My Crazy Moustache:

A PCOS and Reproduction Story

By Angel Rodrigues

Chapter 1

Don't Mock My Crazy Moustache

I am a 5' 4", 270 lbs 38 year old woman and I have a moustache. I also have dry skin patches, irregular periods, hormonal mood swings that keep everybody guessing who's walking into the room and I have Polycystic Ovarian Syndrome/Disorder.

I didn't even know I had PCOS until I was 28 years old. So on my ten-year anniversary of my discovery I write this personal account, because it is now, ten- years later that I know that I am not alone. I am one, part of a larger network of women around the world who also suffer from this disorder. I am not the only one with a moustache.

The past year I have discovered a wealth of information online and a large network of women desperate like myself in various stages of knowledge reaching out to each other. Tired of the isolation, the persecution, the unanswered questions and the blame for things that are beyond our control for the unwanted symptoms of PCOS. Treated with leprosy like flogging, society ridicules the obese woman of society and stops short of stone throwing at the one's that have facial hair. Society is intolerable at any woman who falls short of the Cosmopolitan cover model. Bottom line, we women are mean to each other. While one is crying on the inside out of shame for the symptoms of PCOS that she cannot control, another will come alone and appear socially acceptable and publicly mock that first woman for having facial hair and being overweight, then turn right around and go home to shave her moustache. The hypocrisy is astounding. At its root it is a packed animal mentality. Survival of the fittest and the ones perceived the weakest must be killed off.

One factor that plays into this lack of national awareness is the medical community. The second an obese woman walks into a doctors office it does not matter what she says or does. All that doctor see's is a woman's whole medical history is null and void and any complains she has are irrelevant to the fact that she is obese. All she has to do is loose weight and all of this will go away thinks the doctor. Are they wrong? Not necessarily. They are correct, but the problem with PCOS is that it prevents you from loosing weight and develops a symptom of insulin resistance. Insulin Resistance is a metabolic disorder that prevents your body from processing the sugars in your system and puts the body into a diabetic like state. Your body will be in a constant state of crisis and when your body is in a constant state of crisis, it will hold onto every ounce of nutrients, fat, cholesterol, vitamin, calorie that it intakes. Your body no longer burns the energy it intakes and instead stores it for a long winter's nap. So loosing weight is not an option. So not only are you gaining and storing weight you don't need, but your tired all the time and your hormones are in crisis, your thoughts are all over the place, your skin is a mess, dry and oil at the same time, dry patches and your hair is falling out. Did I mention the moustache and beard? Women most complain about the Hirsutism, abnormal spots of hair growth. Weather it's the obvious moustache, beard or unibrow, PCOS women also can spout hair in places that shouldn't have it, like a breast, shoulder, neck, butt cheek, or anywhere else that seems abnormal. Doctor's do not take any of this into consideration when they see that obese woman walk into the doctor.

The second and maybe most hurtful of all the PCOS symptoms is infertility. Women with PCOS have irregular hormones and period cycles, not to mention a long laundry list of female reproductive issues that come with its symptom list. Everything from endometriosis, cystic fibroids all over their reproductive organs, no egg's for ovulation, egg's not dropping down during ovulation, to an unfriendly uterus. The list is quite endless honestly. So although women like myself can have children with PCOS it requires extraordinary efforts, specialists and sometimes very costly procedures in order to make that motherhood role in life happen. Some may never know that joy and resolve themselves to the fact that it won't happen.

However, not all hope is lost. Along with the fertility doctors that have taken the extra measures to educate themselves on PCOS and how to assist women in that life hurdle, there are other doctors who specialize in PCOS. Some family practitioners have at least become knowledgeable enough to recognize the symptoms to refer out to an endocrinologist who does specialize in it, but once your in that specialists care it is up to the patient to know whether this doctor has the appropriate skill set to treat their PCOS. Some doctors are still, of the mindset that if they just lost weight all would be well. A patient with PCOS will let you know quickly that if she could she would. No woman with PCOS is happy about it and no woman with PCOS would choose to be overweight and struggling in life. A woman with PCOS would like to have a magic pill to make it all right and working correctly. A woman with PCOS would love to shave off her moustache and beard and pluck those few straggler hairs and be done with it. A woman with PCOS would love to skip the electrolysis and go get a pedi instead. A woman with PCOS is just like you women without, but we also know that there are a lot of you that just hide it well. We women struggle enough in life, so instead of making each other's lives that much more difficult, try empathy and compassion. They both are traits that make everyone happy. It does not mean you approve of the disease and accept it, but instead the woman living with its burden.

Chapter 2

I'm Just A Puzzle. Or am I Puzzled? I Forget.

Sometimes it takes getting to the lowest of lows in your mind, heart and soul to see what is truly valuable in your life. Recently I went through a really dark time in my life and allowed myself to feel some kind of way about the people in my life. It wasn't until the reality of it all came crashing down did I strip back the layers to my onion and see what was at the root of it all. I am a hood rat.

I grew up with a single mother in and out of government paid for housing systems. My mother's main income was welfare for many, many years of my life. The windows of her working were very small and usually because we lost welfare for various reasons at that time in our life. So although my mother didn't let me hang outside and mingle with the other hood rats, I was still a hood rat. My mother gave us the perception that we were better than them because we weren't out in the open committing illegal activities or seen in the daylight for what we were, but underneath it all we were no better. She taught me to lie to myself. She taught me that if I believe something strongly enough it makes it so. That when my back is against the wall and I'm exposed to just come out fighting and by any means necessary to make those puzzle pieces fit back into my picture again. To lie. My puzzle was frayed and wrong.

As I grew I realized this puzzle needed smoothing and I worked hard to try and find the right pieces and to make a portrait of myself that didn't look anything like the original picture, but using the same coping skills. I lied, cheated, stole and blamed others in order to keep my perception of my new reality alive and to make my puzzle smooth. I never really got it right and therefore always felt off.

So when recent life events took place and someone who knew the hood rat in me came back into my life and gave me pieces to my puzzle that seemed to fit, I quickly realized that those pieces were to the old picture and I quickly became angry and threw all the pieces on the floor. I did not want those pieces. I did not want that picture that was developing. I did not want to be the hood rat again. I rejected that intrusion and hated myself for even entertaining the thought of having those pieces in my puzzle.

Now I stand here with an incomplete puzzle. I stand here with pieces missing from my identity, slowly but surely I will find the right pieces and not just any piece to put in their place. I am standing here searching my soul and the world that exists for everyone to live in for pieces that make my portrait a masterpiece. I have too many positives in my life for me to take any other approach to all of this. I have too many things to be grateful for and too much love in my life in order to give up on me. I have a circle of protection around me that keeps me safe from those that wish me harm and those that want me in their lives at a cost of giving up what I really love and want in my life. At a cost of myself. No one and nothing is worth having me unless it is part of my life and identity that I am building for myself. I refuse to be a hood rat. I refuse to feed the parts of myself that are rotten, outdated and toxic about myself. So unless you already are in my everyday life and unless you are well aware of your place in my life (my husband, my children, my real friends and you know who you are) then you are nothing to me. You are a discarded puzzle piece.

Chapter 3

I Am Not Ignorant to The Fact That I'm Fat.

When you're faced with the cold, hard fact that you will never be able to produce an offspring, naturally, it can be the thing that makes or breaks you. Off and on throughout my years of womanhood, I was told different things. "It's normal to go months without a period," "it's just how your body works, that's all," and the all too often "stop complaining, some women would love to give up their period's." Yet, when I was married and wanting to have children, the tag lines changed. Now I heard "your barren, its a fact of life and you should seek therapy to deal with it," or "if its meant to happen, it will happen, don't worry about it." Well, I was worried. Very worried as a matter of fact. I went a whole year without a period at one point and my husband and I had been trying to conceive for years. Then I met the one and only doctor with a clue, an endocrinologist, who had become my specialist to get to the root of the problem. Why wasn't I having regular periods?

This doctor asked me seemingly unrelated question after question. Was I growing facial hair? How was my sex drive? Did it hurt to have intercourse? Did I have rough, dry patches of skin on my body? Did I find it hard to loose weight and gain it suddenly and without a change in diet? Did I have mood swings? It was as if the man had been following me around all day long and knew me. I was shocked. He was certain. I had PCOS (Polycystic Ovarian Syndrome). Now, we all have the same reaction to the word syndrome. Yeah, whatever. This is just one of those disease that's going to be a blanket for what you can't figure out - right? Wrong. This disease was called a syndrome, because it was virtually new in the medical community, but not in the gender. Women have been suffering with this disease for so long, that it, like so many other medical complaints by women, was brushed off as, women being women.

Well, this woman was very relieved. Relieved to find out that all of the things that she had been brushing off as just part of her screwed up personality had a name. It was a bona fide disease. I then learned that with some changes to my diet and some minor tinkering from a fertility specialist, I could have kids. I had never felt so happy in my life. I felt, relieved, angry, happy and exhausted all in one felt swoop. I was so angry at all those other doctors who dismissed my complaints and who had brushed aside my longing to be a mother, as a full diaper out of luck story.

Lesson to learn here boys and girls, is that no matter who you are or what you may be feeling, a doctor is not the best indicator of what is going wrong inside the human body. Sure they can read the tests they send you on and they can take the pieces of the puzzle you give them and try to create a picture, but not always do they get the picture right and had pieces missing in order to get the whole picture. It takes a person who takes charge of their own medical care by educating themselves on their own symptoms and possible diagnosis. This can be done on the internet or in a library. If you feel a certain way or have been told certain things from a doctor and don't feel its right or even just want to check just to be sure, its up to you to do so. Write down all your symptoms or diagnosis and look them up. Chances are that you will come up with a list of questions or possibilities that will lead you to the doctor again and if you don't have a great working communication between you and your doctor then you are at the wrong doctor. Get a new one. Yes, its annoying and time consuming, but aren't you worth it? Having PCOS doesn't mean your infertile, but it does mean that you have to advocate for what you want. This may mean that in the end you may not be able to produce an offspring, but will adopt instead. Which is great. So many children in this country are left without a loving home and you could offer that. However, with the right medications and care for your own health with PCOS, you can lessen the chances of developing cysts and the dreaded ovarian cancer that is so common amongst PCOS carriers. A daily dose of birth control sounds like any oxymoron if you can't produce children on your own, but it will keep your plumbing working so to speak. If you keep it working, then there is a lessened chance of cysts developing, because you will be shedding your uterus monthly. Keeping those cells in you is not health, no matter how the medical community wants to cut it. I'm very frightened, as is my fertility doctor by the prospect of permanent infertility for our gender due to the over use of birth controls that only have you shed your uterus every year or five years for some. Our bodies were developed with the idea that monthly shedding is important and there's a reason for that and for women with PCOS this is even more important. Take charge of your own health and don't ever let or keep a doctor who tells you to "just let it go".

How you say? Well, a dog or a seal or some other cute animal can balance a ball on its nose and do so because it has nothing else to think about. I on the other hand can put the ball on my nose, but then have to look down at the cereal being spilled on the couch or the child proof lock being unlocked by a smart ass 3 year old. How am I supposed to diet when I have 100's of things that demand my minute to minute attention? I eat to survive. Nothing more, nothing less. Well, I guess more, in that I use it as a coping skill too. Nothing calms my nerves more than a fancy coffee drink with whipped cream, chocolate drizzle and a hint of mint cooling off my drink of bliss! Or maybe its the homework stress of soda and chips. Or the celebratory sushi meal or seafood extravaganza for passing go and collecting $200! No matter what food is never balanced and neither is the ball on my nose.

This isn't to say I am free of blame, because obviously that is a lie. I do love salad, vegetables, lean meats and cheeses. I just love food! However, it is up to me to care enough about myself to care what I put in me. I make damn sure the kids eat well, but when it comes to me, well ya, not so much. Of course this falls upon my husband too. He eats what I eat. He and I agree, a diet is necessary, but as a lifestyle change. We should be able to eat what we want, in moderation, but with more exercise. I agree, but when I have 2 papers due in 24 hours and I am bogged down by life, a crying sick kid, twin tantrums and a weird infestation of flies from the neighborhood community garden, I just want a damn potato chip!

My hormones are in a nightmarish hell right now, PCOS is really kicking my ass and most days I just have to accept that....

....this fatty wanker is struggling.....

Chapter 4

I'm a Medical Mystery.

No matter what I do, the adage damned if I do, damned if I don't really applies here. I can have all the best intentions to be healthier, but my body always chooses to poop out on me when I need it the most. I have the weirdest thyroid ever, that even baffles the doctors. I am as usual a medical mystery!

See when I was pregnant with the twins I developed a lump in my right thyroid and it was undiagnosed until some months afterwards when I was knee deep into postpartum depression that a doctor discovered it. It should have been caught while twins were in utero, but that's another story... I will get to that one at some point. So anyway, the lump was too small to biopsy, but just big enough to screw up my whole system. Fast forward to now (3 1/2 years later) and that lobe of my thyroid either shuts off or rains hormones and floods my system. So I fluctuate between hyperthyroidism to hypothyroidism. It's a nightmare. Some days I'm exhausted, confused, overwhelmed and my body aches something horrible! Other days I have the energy of 1,000 men, I'm the smartest woman in the world, I am dropping mad weight and I am enduring heart palpitations that make me feel like I ran a marathon. It really is insane! I am a walking medical mystery!

So needless to say, even my doctor said "Its not a wonder you can't loose weight....your body doesn't know if its coming or going." I laugh and say, yes I know the feeling. I am truly a medical mystery!

Chapter 5

Screw You Doctor!

When I was told by doctor after doctor after doctor that I would "never" be able to conceive a child on my own, not only was I depressed, but empty inside, literally. I started to blame myself, my gene's, my choices, my everything. I was going through all the emotions that a woman does when she is faced with infertility. Then everything changed.

I used Clomid and had my first child in 2005. A beautiful, smart, perfect little boy. Then we wanted him to have a sibling. So Clomid round two came and nothing and so we decided to give it one more shot and there they were, my twin baby boys in 2008. Also born beautiful, perfect and as exciting and new as the first baby. So we were now a family of 5 and we were complete. Or so we thought.

Then comes 2009 and nature takes its course. One fine week in March I thought I had the stomach flu. I had just started a job after being a stay at home mom for 3 years and was ready to go back to work. I kept throwing up and had this fluttering feeling in my stomach and was so tired. Then one day the light bulb went on over my head and I thought, "duh, maybe I should take a pregnancy test, even though I know it will be negative, but just maybe." So I did and much to my disbelief and shock, there they were. The two lines telling me I was positively pregnant. I handed my son the stick and told him to run to daddy. He did and we all stood there in shock. Even though my son had no idea why we were shocked. So still not believing it, I had my husband stay home with twins and I took my oldest with me to the hospital (my doctor was closed) to have a quick pee test. They too confirmed the first test and declared me pregnant. I was a perfectly 7 week along pregnant woman.

Fast forward to week 18 and the sono that we pregnant women all wait for, to find out the gender. It is a girl! We both could not believe it. I cried like I did for the first sono and the second. All three pregnancies carrying with it it's own shock, individually and as a blessing. So I am here as a testament to the fact that even PCOS as a diagnosis does not mean your infertile. Sometimes have to use the gifts that medical science gave us to teach our bodies what to do. I firmly believe that my body didn't know what to do and with a little Clomid, I taught my body how to do what should have come naturally. As evolution comes into our lives, sometimes the natural evolution of our own bodies and cycles that exist, leave us. We are also accustomed to living life on our own terms and on our own time table's. So when things don't happen as quickly as we wish or in the way that we wish we forced them to happen. Which is fine, but is also a life lesson to teach us to slow down and live life as it is intended. Naturally.

Chapter 6

Vaginal Delivery: What Really Happens!

When I was having my first child, I was completely unprepared for what was about to take place "down there". I have since had 4 deliveries. A singleton, a set of twins and lastly a singleton. I am what the OB/GYN community calls "a pro". Not of course in the Michelle Duggar sense, but needless to say I know what I'm doing by now. So after our recent delivery of our fourth and final child, I realized something. There was a ton of mom's in labor and delivery with me that were terrified, having panic attacks and uncooperative with the nurses, causing long deliveries and unnecessary C-sections, because patience was wearing thin on all parties.

I say unnecessary, because if someone had just explained not only what was going on, but how to deal with it, they might have calmed the mother to be down and eliminated the tense muscles in her bottom that were causing baby to stay inside, probably terrified of what was going on. Mother after mother was offered (including myself) "Valium" and "Morphine," to "ease delivery". I'm sorry, but what?!? Did I just hear that right? Mother after mother being drugged instead of taught how to deliver. I realized that I had my first 3 children in a different state and with different tact's of labor and delivery, but come on. Is medicinal applications during labor and delivery regional?

I am now assuming yes and have decided to write this article, so that it may be universal and maybe save some mother and baby from having to drug themselves up and maybe cut up, when all they needed to do was focus and relax.

First of all, no one bothers to tell you that pushing a baby out of your vagina, means mentally telling your body to push with your rear end. Pretty much like trying have a very large bowel movement and your constipated. Even though you have been taught your whole life and during your whole pregnancy not to do that, as it will cause Hemorroids, this is what you need to do, to push a baby out. If you mentally use all your power to push what you think is something out of your vagina, you will get no where fast. Going against all of your mental programming is also the certainty that you will not only "fart," but "have a bowel movement" on the nurses and doctors and whom ever else is in the room, which is the thee most unlady like thing you can do, or so your programmed to think.

During this undetermined amount of time and pain, you will essentially be mentally overriding all that you know and trying to get your mind and body to work in harmony to have the largest bowel movement every, no matter what comes out of your body, in the presence of strangers, family and whom ever else you invite to this event. The result will be a baby! I promise.

Then you also have to mentally prepare yourself for the feeling of pushing a baby out of your vagina, even though you are trying to think about pushing something out of your bum. Epidural or not, you are going to feel this. The epidural may help with contractions and such, but if you are in the pushing stage, the strong desire to push and get it over with will override the epidural. So you have to prepare yourself for this. I liken it to when you have a gut wrenching intestinal bug and you really need to go to the bathroom and everything in your body is working to squeeze that bug out of your intestines. You cannot do anything, but roll with it. Your whole body will role with a contraction that will vibrated from rib all the way down your thighs and that sensation to push whatever or in this case whom ever out of your body will overwhelm you.

You will then have to take in a deep breath (so not to pass out) and put your chin to your chest, grab your legs by the thighs and pull them up towards you and push mentally in your bum to get rid of this feeling. Then you will start to feel a burning sensation in your vaginal area. It is the baby's head pushing its way out. Now some women have episiotomies and I have not had to have one of these, so if you do need this, I am sorry, I cannot offer any first hand information on this matter. I have had the luck of several great nurses who spend the time, while I'm pushing, to stretch the peri-vaginal region with their gloved fingers, to help assist in the stretching of that skin for baby not to tear me.

So as I was saying, this burning that comes with baby stretching the vagina for exit, then mentally clashes with all that you are trying to program your body to do at the time and you really need to maintain focus and perseverance, otherwise you will suck that baby back up and all efforts are lost. With all this focus, keep trying to push out of your bum, keep the method of tucking chin, pulling legs, taking deep breath's and ignoring all things that are coming out of your bum at the time, all while hoping it is over soon. Essentially, your a plate spinner. Keep it all going and you are good. You will be exhausted on all fronts and people are standing around looking at you in all your glory. The pressure is overwhelming, but you have to be able to shut it all out.

Then the moment comes. You know you are one or two pushes away from that baby coming out and just then everyone tells you to stop and hold it. Hold it! Did they just say stop!?! You want to scream and beat someone up, but you are too busy trying not to let go of what is the head of your baby trying to emerge. For you it will be like trying to hold in a bad taco from a bar in Mexico. You hear the doctor being called, but then they arrive and you have to wait for them to put their gloves on, put cover up's on all parts (because god forbid they get dirty) and just in time to catch the baby (you hope) and take all the credit for delivery. Even though all the nurses did all the work of delivery and you did all the work of labor. I say give the mom and nurses the doctor's paycheck and we can all over look this little discrepancy.

Now a little more on that head emerging. Once the head emerges, you are not done. The relief that comes with that head coming out is enough for you to relax for a second, but then comes the shoulders which for some can be more painful that the head itself. Then the rest of the baby comes out and all you feel is a squishy, slimy, quick moving object pass through and your whole bottom region is screaming in relief and burning from stretching. You finally stop gripping the bars on the bedside and you can stop trying to spin those plates, but just then the doctor lets you know they are going to deliver (or you hope they tell you) the placenta. They do this while they clean your baby and you wait to hear the cry of the living, human being created by you and your partner.

The feeling of the placenta being delivered was dependent on the doctor that delivered. The first one was screamingly painful, uncomfortable and similar to ripping of a scab on a large wound, when it wasn't ready. I cried. Then for my twins, I had to go through it twice. It was very similar to the first one, but lessened in strength, but hated just as much. Then with my fourth and final one, I can honestly say I felt it very lightly. The doctor took his time taking the placenta from my uterus and did it in small steps until it detached and then he delivered it, which felt like a big, glob of slimy gum coming out of my vagina. Gross, but that is what it was like. Then the after affects of my epidural kicked in and I shook and teeth chattered until it was out of my system.

With your baby in your arms and at different points being cared for and checked out by nurses, your body will undergo a lot of changes. If you had an epidural, once that is out of your system, your body is then beginning the healing process. It will be sore and foreign to you for some time afterwards. I'm sure this process is different for every woman. The nurses will give you numbing stuff for your vaginal care and stool softeners to help you move them. Your body is in shock essentially and not only are you going to be mentally afraid to have a bowel movement, but your body is swollen and all out of whack. Your uterus will be contracting to go back to normal size and you will be bleeding and urinating all over the place until that heals. The urinating on yourself varies in amount of time for healing, but takes the full 6 weeks usually to be back to its pre-baby self and for some of us, not even then. The bleeding depends on how long it takes for your uterus to heal. Usually within 24 hours the stool softeners will help you with the bowel movement and the nurses will expect you to empty your bladder shortly after giving birth and if you are like me, you had a catheter during delivery (various reasons) and you will urinate blood for a while and it will burn, but if you don't urinate on your own, they will take it from you, via catheter again.

Not to mental all the blood pressure readings and baby monitoring during delivery, they do one last check of temps and blood pressures before heading you and baby off to recovery with baby. All in all, this whole process will leave your vagina sore, swollen, bruised and in some serious need for a day at the spa. So take care of yourself and take care of your vagina, because we all know you will need it again. Follow doctors orders and wait the 6 weeks before engaging in any activity that requires insertion of anything in there. Not only for bacteria reasons during healing, but also because you want the vagina to heal fully and not be the stretched out cave that we all fear will happen once we deliver a child from there. Pre-baby vagina is just around the corner, just don't be in a rush to get there.

Vaginal delivery can be a happy, productive, drug free (give or take an epidural) experience, but it is up to the mom to be informed and in control. Don't allow fear or medical degree's get in the way of what is to be a positive, loving experience for you and baby. Your vagina will thank you later.

Chapter 7

Postpartum Depression

No one talks about dealing with postpartum depression when you're a woman living with PCOS. No one has any answers for you. Postpartum Depression is difficult for the medical community to understand as it is, much less coupled with a disease no one really understands to its fullest extent. One chief question I had when dealing with it was: when exactly does postpartum depression go away? When I was pregnant with my first, it took about 6 months. However, with twins, does that mean it takes twice as long? They're just over 5 months now and I love them dearly, but I am so depressed that I'm pretty sure my absent mindedness of my own personal care is a symptom of the depression and not sleep deprivation. How do I overcome it? How do I find the special things that gets every mom through the day? How do I find that special something that makes a mom snap out of her postpartum and say to herself "Oh, wow! Look at this perfect little angel that has come from my husband and myself. I so love being a mom." When does that come? Because right now, I'm so not feeling it.

Supposedly 10% of all pregnancies are plagued with Postpartum Depression (Source: excerpt from Postpartum Depression Fact Sheet: NWHIC). Yet it appears as though that the number should be much larger. That 10% only includes mom's who sought help from a medical professional and who fit a certain criteria for PPD.

When I talk to other mom's they all express some degree larger or smaller that could fall into some spectrum of what most of us would classify as PPD. However, with Baby Blues being the lesser end of depression after delivery and being the most common, unless your on the extreme opposite end of PPD, where a death occurs for the infant, most of the PPD suffers aren't classified and included in the 10% statistic. As a self diagnosed suffer of PPD, I knew I wasn't alone, but that didn't make me feel any better.

I wanted to be in love with my babies. I wanted to showcase them like the bookend babies that they were. I felt robbed. Robbed of the most important part of having a baby, the precious moments after delivery when you get to know each other outside of the scary ultrasound pictures and middle the night kick sessions. Instead what I got was a creeping feeling that came over me every time they were near me. I didn't want to hear them cry, I didn't want to look at them, I didn't want to hold them or feed them. I did of course, out of necessity and a desire to have them live and be around when the dust settled. I did it because I'm sure deep down I loved them and all their infinite loveliness, but for the first 5 months, I so wasn't feeling it.

Looking for some relief from the dark hole I felt that I fell into, I naturally turned to my husband. My support system, my rock. He didn't understand. He hadn't been through it and he didn't know what to do for me or with me for that matter. He just worked more. I was home alone with my toddler and newborn twins. We had just moved out of state and I knew no one. I had one friend that visited every now and then from a 3 hour away trip, but that was it. The little family we do have lived 4 states away. I was alone, depressed, in high demand and unsure of how to deal with it. I had never cried so much as I did in the first 5 months of my twins lives. They cried all the time. I knew they had colic and colic meant crying, but one of twins was also throwing up all the time and he was loosing his voice. I took them to the emergency room, he had acid reflux. Now I had newborns with colic, one with acid reflux and a toddler who wanted his mommy. Daddy was at work all the time and I couldn't even shower without something going wrong. I had to take charge and gain control over myself and my situation.

I started talking my vitamins everyday, with an extra dose of B12 and B6, mood lifters. I had stopped taking my prenatal's when I learned I couldn't breast feed. I started eating better and getting out of the house in small bursts. I started setting up play stations for my toddler and giving him chores and activities to keep him busy. I found that music and dancing helped not only distract the babies from crying, even if only for a few minutes, but also got me laughing and smiling again.

My twins were now 6 months old and after a full month of forcing myself to get up, join in and participate, my PPD started to lift. It really is just that, a feeling that the dark cloud that you were living in, just lifts off of you and the sun comes out. Even if by coincidence, that the PPD lifted at that time because its time was up or because of my forced participation in life, the result is the same – happiness.

Becoming a mother was a choice, but no one chooses PPD. It chooses you. Knowing your a statistic, only gives a name to the problem, but its up to you how you deal with that problem. No different than living with PCOS. My heart goes out to those mothers who have no choice and end up in the extreme end of PPD and a death occurs. I wonder how many of them were also double battling PPD and PCOS and were undiagnosed. Before becoming a mother, I was one of societies rock throwers at their crime. Now having dealt with a fraction of the pain they go through I can only hurt for them. I would like to think that if I was not so determined to be happy again and lost sight of what was important I would have sought professional help and kept myself from going to such an extreme, but who knows? Everyday women have children and deal with PPD in one extreme or another, but it doesn't have to be a lost cause and rob you of the love a newborn and mother have for each other. Professional services are out there and PPD is a legitimate and life saving reason to seek it. Feel good about yourself and your little gift, if your dealing with PPD, get help. Your both work it.

Chapter 8

Fear of Delivery

Fear. This is the one thing that has been a common thread throughout my whole first pregnancy. Fear that I would loose the baby after so much time nurturing him in my womb. Fear that he would be born without all of the standard baby equipment, i.e. arms, legs, eyes, feet. I feared one thing above and beyond all of these very realistic, but improbably outcomes of my 9 month journey. I feared the final departure. The exit. How in the world was an expected 6 pound baby going to come out of the womb that carried him so lovingly for the past 9 months?

I knew that countless, brave woman had endured what I was about to embark on and lived to tell about it. However, there are also countless, brave women who died in child birth. Even as recent as the week before my deliver, in the same hospital. How was I to be any different? However, the one fear that crept over me like someone walking on a grave, was the thought that the baby was going to have to come out. More importantly, come out of there!

During the last week of my pregnancy I was diagnosed with Pre-Eclampsia and Toxemia. My blood pressure readings were around 201/199. I was swollen and my skin had a layer of water underneath it, giving me the appearance of a walking waterbed. It was great for my pregnancy self esteem. Pregnancy is beautiful! Right?

After I was admitted to the hospital 6 days before my due date, the doctor's wanted to induce. I went through rounds of medications, on a constant drip. Pitocin, Magnesium, Cervical Monitors, the whole kit and kaboodle. My blood pressure was so high that I had very little sight left and my eyes were black all the way around them. I was miserable. I was ready for an epidural. Once all of the contractions were bearable and I could lay still and rest, it came back. The thought. The thought that my baby was coming and he was coming out of there.

Three days had gone by and all the medical efforts weren't making my baby stand and deliver. I firmly believed it was because he could hear my thoughts. The fear of the inevitable. He knew I was terrified of him coming out and splitting me in two, leaving him alone with his equally as terrified father, with his own paternal fears. So he kicked back and relaxed. What else was there to do?

Then just as everybody decided to let my body relax and I could finally eat real food, my water broke. I started to cut into my eggplant parmesan, when I thought I peed myself. The nurse tested my waters and confirmed that I was indeed labor and not incontinent. I was so upset that I couldn't eat, I wanted to cry, but I think I used them all up during the contractions.

So I just lie there and sulked until they hit. They! The all encompassing, body quaking, earth shattering contractions. The natural way your body gets you prepared for the event about to take place. It's kind of like the alarm that sounds when there's a fire and all the fire people come running out and rush to the fire. Yeah, that's the type of enthusiasm that goes into each contraction. Your not sure if their ever going to end or if they will be the death of you.

I was inclined to think they were going to be the death of me. In other words, I was pretty much of the mind set that either me or the baby wasn't going to make it out alive and instead of my husband standing by my side looking at me lovingly, he should be out planning a funeral. Morbid? Yes, but this is what fear does to a person. It robs you of the enjoyment of some of the most wonderful things in life.

Until that wonderful conclusion comes and you sit there, looking into the babies eyes. Him/her looking back at you. Checking to see if he or she was issued all of the standard equipment and you want to just sigh in relief. So you do. Then you realize, you were just afraid of becoming a mother. Then you are one and your grateful, scared, relieved, petrified and elated all in one joyous moment. The baby came out of there and guess what? You both made it. Both in tact, hopefully and without even thinking about it, you will do it again.

Chapter 9

Why Not Get Two Out at One Whack?

I was only six weeks pregnant and I knew something was unusual. I had my first child two years prior to this and even though I wrote down every minute detail, my mind was certain. This one was definitely different. Like so many women in modern society, infertility was the mysterious white elephant in the room when it came to the question of motherhood. I took Clomid (a common infertility drug) and I was off and running. Blood test after blood test, I learned that the HcG (pregnancy hormone) levels were doubling by the day and was well over the levels of my first pregnancy. I became suspicious. My husband became excited. He so wanted twins. As he claimed "why not get two out at one whack?"

Then there they were. My sonogram showed what I had suspected. Two jumping grains of rice. I wanted to name one Uncle Ben and the other Long Grain.

I wanted to name one Uncle Ben and the other Long Grain. At each check point in my pregnancy I became riddled with anxiety until it was confirmed in some medical manner that I was still pregnant with twins. Fear of a miscarriage, one baby squishing the other or the lining of my uterus "absorbing" the baby as the baby books called it.

Every rational, probable, irrational and highly unlikely outcome of my pregnancy plagued me the night before every pending check point. Then 8 months into my pregnancy I hit the wall. My body was done. Stick a fork in my behind, because this turkey was ready to carve. I wanted to scream into my vagina, okay, guys you can get out now. Well, if I could even see that part of me at that point. I would have been happy just to see my swollen, sausage toes while standing.

At this check point the doctor said that even though I had been experiencing contractions, my body had no other signs of labor. What was I to do now? The babies didn't want to leave and my body had called it quits. I couldn't stand for too long. I couldn't sit for too long. Laying down was murder on my back. Sleep was non existent and I couldn't remember the last time I ate without my esophagus burning like I was the latest fire eating attraction at a circus.

When I saw the sonogram at week 32, I gasped in horror. One baby was standing on the other one's face and smooshing it into my cervix! There was absolutely no room left. I'm pretty sure my organs packed their bags and headed for the nearest exit. I was miserable. My reflection in the mirror was screaming at me to shed all the weight, water, acne, dark circles and mood swings that had been plaguing it for the past 8 months. I'm pretty sure I heard the mirror say "check please"!

So during week 36's check point, I expressed to my doctor how I was done and was unable to carry on. She agreed and sent me to the hospital. There I was, the night before my birthday. My legs spread wide open, they broke my water. Now it was on like Donkey Kong. My contractions were unrelenting.

Unlike my first pregnancy where there was an ebb and flow to them, this time there was no ebb, just flow. On the monitor I could see them go off the chart and never really go back down to a point of relaxing. I wanted an epidural. What I didn't ask for was the reaction to the epidural that almost sent me packing. My blood pressure crashed, I became very cold, shaken and the room went dark. I heard someone say "get the adrenaline," but not much else.

I looked around and saw only nurses. My husband was across the room, to stay out of the way. I was alone and dying. Then like a cannonball making its exit, I was up and out of the darkness. I was warm and scared. I started to cry. The nurse explained everything to me and reassured me the babies weren't harmed. I had no choice but to believe her. I wanted to hold them, on the outside.

Being determined to deliver vaginally, for fear of caring for my twins, my two year old and myself after a cesarean, I kept telling my belly to "get into position boys, were ready for lift off." Eight hours later, baby number one, as he was so lovingly referred to by everybody, made his way out. Then an hour and two minutes later, baby number two, also lovingly called by everybody, came. He was significantly bigger than the first. That's not supposed to happen.

All the baby books and medical staff told me that the bigger one comes out first and that way baby number two is an easier delivery. Oh no, not me. Of course not. I always manage to do things the hard way. But then I saw them and it was all good.

Weighing in at 5.75 lbs and 6.02 lbs, my two grains of rice were larger than most twins, separated in delivery time longer than most twins and not delivered in a cesarean as most twins. I knew it was an unusual pregnancy from the start. Being born on my birthday, giving me the biggest and best birthday present ever. I was running off of an adrenalin high. I was up and walking around right after the delivery and caring for myself and them for the remainder of my stay and up until now. Without blinking an eye.

Now don't get me wrong. I have shed many tears and screamed on the top of my lungs in frustration, but caring for them and seeing their developmental rewards has been the most rewarding experience of my life. Seeing them play with each other and hold each other is the best. Each one so different from each other, but with their own special bond that no one can ever take away from them or me.

Chapter 10

Inspired by Me.

Ask me at various times in my life who I am and you will get a different answer. Not because I am unsure if who I am or a poser, but instead because I am forever growing.

Today is no different. As a woman in the modern world I am very well aware of the confines that are put on me because of my gender, my health issues, societal constructs, and what is expected from me with equal fortitude. I have always tested those boundaries. I wanted to know what was on the other side of the fence. What happens if I ... Yet none of the answers I got brought me any genuine clarity. I got results and answers of course but they were stock answers, pulled from a hat like a rabbit. I had always assumed that those answers were all there was. However with equal excitement to finding out Starbucks had a off the menu menu, I found life has an off the menu menu. There were more options than choosing from column A column b and finally one from column C. Fanfriggtastic!

So now that my options are endless and no longer defined by you, the media's, my favorite song, or even a previous version of myself I truly feel enlightened. I get Buddha and that fortune cookie from fourth grade. I get which way the wind blows and how to survive a zombie evasion. I get it. I am enlightened. I am my own guiding star. I inspire me.

Luckily my path is not walked alone. My soul mate, kindred spirit and life walker, my husband gets it too. He is my spirit animal. Blessed is not just a Christian term, but a feeling and I am living proof that a life can be blessed. Don't let PCOS define you. Don't let infertility define you. Don't let your parents, siblings, friends, past, perceptions, the media, the neighbors, the stranger in line at the grocery store define you. You define you.

You decide what makes you happy, sad, indifferent, ambitious, defeated and everything in between. It is when people stop looking to others for answers do they really find enlightenment. Inspire yourself and rock that crazy moustache!

www.ingramcontent.com/pod-product-compliance
Lightning Source LLC
Chambersburg PA
CBHW070940290526
45795CB00003B/1089